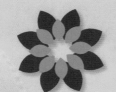

developed by a survivor

for survivors to help

regain mobility and

improve quality of life.

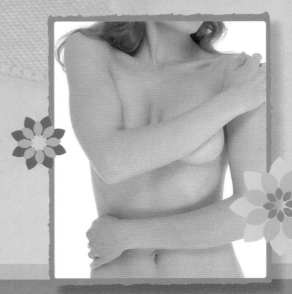

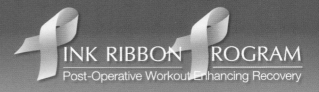
PINK RIBBON PROGRAM
Post-Operative Workout Enhancing Recovery

www.pinkribbonprogram.com

This exercise manual is for those who have had surgery for breast cancer. Exercise is an important part of your treatment and recovery. It will provide restoration of movement in your affected arm and shoulder, improve functional ability in day to day activities and improve your overall well-being.

Everyone is different and heals at her/his own pace. Talk to your doctor or another healthcare team member before starting this or any exercise program. The Pink Ribbon Program works in conjunction with your doctor's recommendations for an exercise program. You may also use this program in conjunction with or as a follow-up program to any prescribed physical therapy.

There are four phases to The Pink Ribbon Program. Each phase should be maintained for two weeks. The progression from one phase to the next will depend on how you are feeling. You can participate in these exercises two to three times per week. Once you have completed this program, you are now ready to join in many types of mainstream activities. Please be aware of any ongoing limitation you may have due to your surgeries.

These exercises can be done as soon as your doctor gives you permission.

GENERAL GUIDELINES

- ❧ You will feel some tightness in your chest and armpit after surgery. This is normal and the tightness will decrease as you continue with The Pink Ribbon Program.
- ❧ Wear comfortable, loose clothing when doing the exercises.
- ❧ Be sure to breathe as you perform each exercise.
- ❧ Due to nerve ending irritation, you many experience burning, tingling or numbness on the arm or chest wall. This is normal. Rubbing or stroking the area with your hand or a soft cloth can help "desensitize" the area.
- ❧ Notify your doctor if you experience unusual swelling or tenderness.

This program is suitable whether your surgery was recent or several years ago and accommodates all fitness levels.

ABOUT THE FOUNDER

Doreen Puglisi, MS is the Founder and Program Director for The Pink Ribbon Program. As an exercise physiologist, Doreen is dedicated to design and implementation of specialty programs for clients with specific medical limitation. While working with patients who were breast cancer survivors, Doreen saw a need to design a specific post-operative program for these survivors. Hence, The Pink Ribbon Program was created. This need became even more apparent when she, herself, was diagnosed with breast cancer. Proactive in her own recovery, Doreen used The Pink Ribbon Program to regain strength, range of motion and a sense of wellbeing that had been lost due to her surgeries. Doreen is the Chairperson of the Health Education and Exercise Science Department at County College of Morris, New Jersey. She holds a Master's degree in Exercise Science and a B.A. from Seton Hall University. Most recently Doreen was invited to Australia where she conducted a nationwide breast cancer awareness campaign sponsored by The National Breast Cancer Foundation. She travels extensively throughout the United States in an effort to train as many health professionals to become certified Pink Ribbon Program instructors so that they can reach out to as many breast cancer survivors as possible.

Preparation

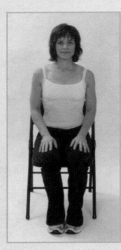

Starting Position:

Seated on a chair

Breathing
Inhale deeply for 4 slow counts, then **exhale** for 4 counts.

Continue for 3-4 repetitions.

As you lengthen through your spine, it should feel like you have a string attached to the crown of the head and your spine is gently being elongated toward the ceiling. At this point, check to see that your ribcage is directly over your hips, your shoulders over your ribcage.

Shoulder Rolls

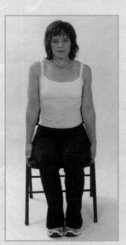
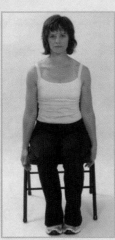

Gently roll the shoulders forward and back, allowing the upper back to release slightly as you do so.

Neck Stretch
Tension Release

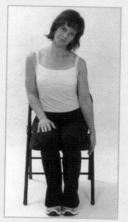 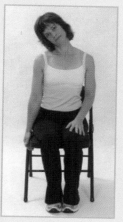 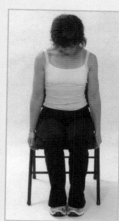

- Allow your head to drop gently to the left, to the right, and then to the front.

- Repeat 2-3 times.

NOTE: Please do not drop the head back. This is considered unsafe.

Abdominal Connection

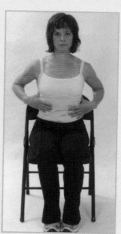

- Place your hands on your abs and imagine that they are a corset.

- **Inhale**.

- As you exhale, gently contract your abdominals. It should feel as though you are bracing yourself for a punch in the abdominal area.

- Try to breathe comfortably for 3-4 breaths while maintaining this abdominal connection.

1 Seated Shoulder Slides

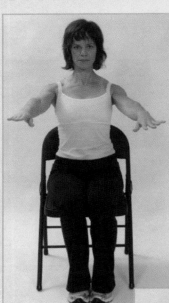

Starting Position:

Seated on chair, neutral pelvis with arms reaching out in front of you.

❧ **Inhale –** Draw the scapula (shoulder blades) together without arching the back.
Exhale – return to neutral.

❧ **Inhale –** Sliding the scapula apart, feel as if your fingertips are being pulled away from you. Keep the collarbone wide. Be careful not to elevate the shoulders.

❧ Repeat 3-4 times.

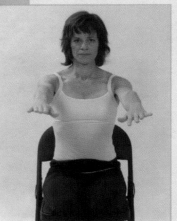

FOCUS: Protraction & retraction of the scapula/ scapula stabilization

NOTES:

_____

_____

2 Open Elbows

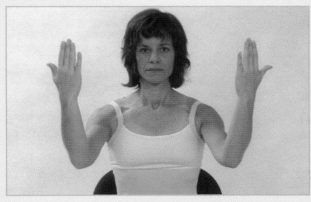

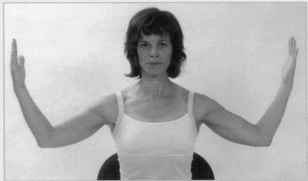

Starting Position:

Seated on chair, neutral pelvis, raise arms out in front of you, palms facing ceiling. Bend the elbow to 90 degrees. Elbows raised to slightly below shoulder height, palms facing you. **Inhale** to stay.

ର **Exhale.**

ର Open arms as wide as possible keeping elbows bent. Try not to allow the ribcage to move forward in space. Do not elevate shoulders. **Inhale –** Return to start position.

ର Repeat 3-4 times.

FOCUS: Scapula stabilization, horizontal shoulder abduction, chest expansion

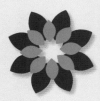

NOTES:

_____

_____

3 Overhead Stretch

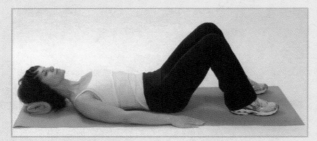

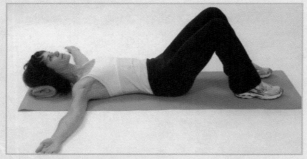

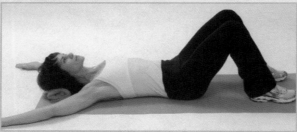

Starting Position:

Lying supine (face up) with knees bent, arms by side, palms facing the floor.

- **Inhale** and slide arms along the floor. As your arms reach 90 degrees (T position), turn palms up to face the ceiling. Slide as high as you can.

- **Exhale –** Slide your arms back down by your side, rotating the palms to face the floor.

- Repeat 3-4 times.

NOTE: Try to keep your shoulder blades on the floor; do not rotate your torso. Use the floor as support for the weight of your arms.

FOCUS: Scapula stabilization, abduction with external rotation of shoulder

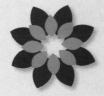

NOTES:

_____

_____

_____

4 Supine Arm Circles

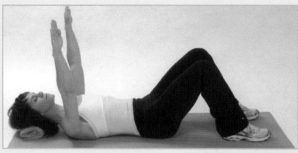

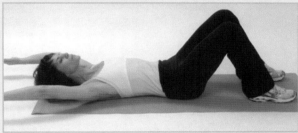

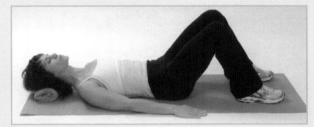

Starting Position:

Lying supine (face up) with knees bent, arms by your side, reach both arms up to the ceiling, palms facing away from you. (perpendicular to the floor.)

- **Exhale –** Reach both arms overhead as far as they will reach comfortably.

- **Inhale.**

Slowly return both arms to a 90 degree angle of shoulder flexion with fingertips reaching toward the ceiling.

- **Exhale –** Return arms by your side.

- Repeat 3-4 times.

NOTE: Be sure to keep the ribcage relaxed, keep the midback on the mat, and keep the collarbone wide.

FOCUS: Scapula stabilization while moving through shoulder flexion/extension

NOTES:

_____

_____

5 Arm Scissors

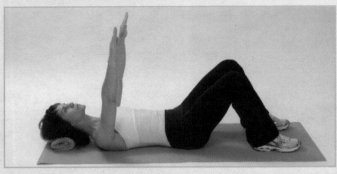

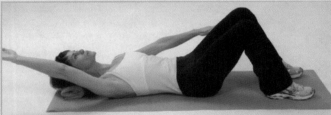

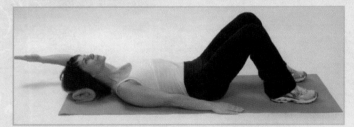

Starting Position:

Lying supine (face up) with knees bent, arms reaching to the ceiling (perpendicular to the floor), palms facing each other. **Inhale** to stay.

- **Exhale –** Reach one arm directly overhead, while the other arm reaches down toward the feet.
  Inhale – Return to start position.

- **Exhale –** Reach the other arm overhead, while the opposite arm reaches down toward the feet.
  Inhale – Return to start position.

- Repeat 3-4 times.

NOTE: Be sure to keep the ribcage relaxed, keep the midback on the mat, collarbone wide.

NOTES:

_____

_____

6 Supine Puppet

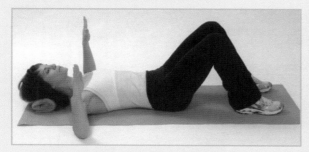

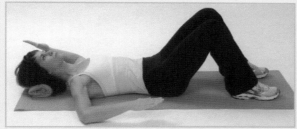

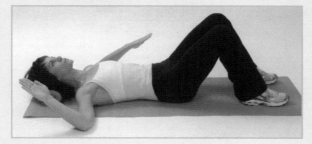

Starting Position:

Lying supine with knees bent, arms out to sides (T position), just below shoulder height; bend elbows to 90 degrees, with fingertips pointing to ceiling. **Inhale** to stay.

☙ **Exhale –** Keeping your elbows and upper arm on the floor – internally rotate the right arm – this is done at the shoulder joint so that the hand moves forward, toward the floor and the palm faces the floor.

☙ At the same time, externally rotate the left arm – this is done at the shoulder joint so that the hand moves backwards and the palm faces up to the ceiling. Move to a comfortable range of motion.

☙ **Inhale –** Return to the starting position. **Exhale –** Reverse the action.

☙ Repeat 3-4 times.

NOTE: It is not necessary for the hand to reach the floor. Move within a comfortable range of motion.

FOCUS: Internal/external rotation at shoulder joint, scapula stabilization

NOTES:

_____

_____

7 Seated Rock 'n' Roll (C- Curve)

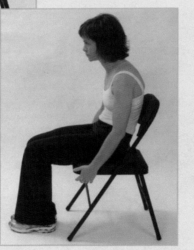

Starting Position:

Seated on a chair or mat: **Inhale,** grow taller.

ॐ **Exhale –** Contract your abdominals and roll slightly back of your sit bones.

ॐ **Inhale –** Use your abs to come back onto your sit bones.

ॐ Repeat 5-6 times.

FOCUS: Lower back flexion and abdominal connection

DEFINITION: The sit bones are the ischial tuberosity, to be exact. They are quite literally the bones under the flesh of the butt that you sit on.

NOTES:

_____

_____

_____

8 Rotation

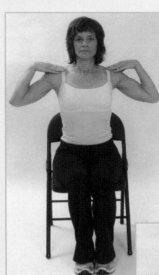

Starting Position:

Seated on a chair or mat, pelvis neutral, both hands on head or on shoulders (whichever range of motion allows). **Inhale** to stay.

- **Exhale –** Rotate as far as possible to the right.
- **Inhale –** Come back to center.
- Reverse direction.
- Repeat 3-4 times.

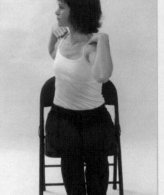

NOTE:
Draw your navel toward your spine and rotate from your waist. Keep your hips pointing forward. Remember to rotate up and out of your hips.

FOCUS:
Core stability and trunk rotation

NOTES:

_____

_____

_____

9 Lateral Flexion

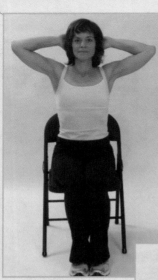

Starting Position:

Seated on chair, pelvis neutral, both hands on head or on shoulders (whichever range of motion allows). **Inhale**.

∝ **Exhale** – Laterally bend your upper body to the right (bend body at the waist, to the right), keeping both sit bones down.

∝ **Inhale** – Return to vertical. **Exhale** – Reverse direction. **Inhale** – Return to vertical.

∝ Repeat 3-4 times.

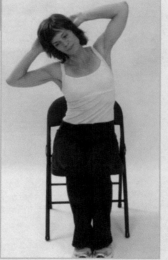

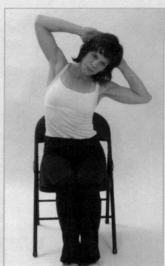

NOTE:
Come up and over the hips. Do not sink down. Expand the ribs that face the ceiling.

NOTES:

_____

_____

_____

Mermaid Stretch

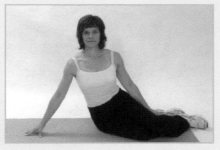
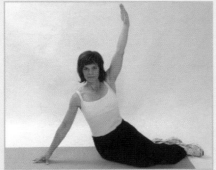
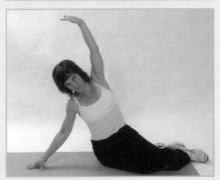

Starting Position:

Sitting on the right hip with both legs folded to the left. The right hand is on the floor for support. Keep your left shoulder down as you extend your left arm up toward the ceiling. Bring the inside of your arm as close to your ear without hiking up your shoulder.

- Keep your left hip grounded as you lengthen your spine and the stretch moves up through the center of your body. Extend your spine so far up that you have nowhere left to go with the stretch but to take it over to the side. Do not let your ribs pop forward as you curve to the side.

- Your support hand moves further away from your body to increase the stretch. You can also fold the supporting elbow down onto the floor. Keep your shoulders down and your scapula settled in your back, even at the farthest point of your reach.

- To initiate your return, send your left sit bone down toward the mat. Then use your abs to begin to bring your torso up to a vertical position.

NOTE: Stay flat. Do not let your back arch, your ribs pop out, or your shoulder twist inward.

Keep your shoulders down and your scapula engaged on your back.

The head moves as an extension of the spine.

The whole stretch should feel good.

NOTES:

_____

_____

11 Arm Circles Supine

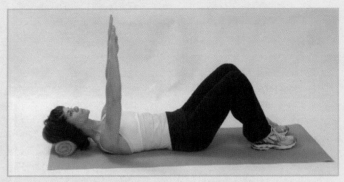

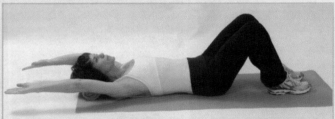

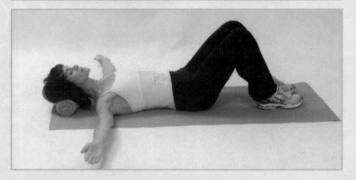

Starting Position:

Lying supine with knees bent, arms by your side. **Inhale –** reach the arms up and then overhead.

- **Exhale –** Circle the arms around and down towards the hips, returning to start position.

- Repeat 3-4 times, then reverse direction.

FOCUS: Scapula stabilization and full range of motion at the shoulder joint

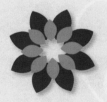

NOTES:

_____

_____

_____

12 Touchdown

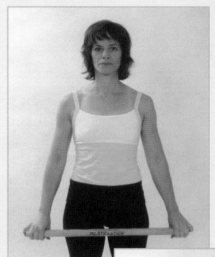

Starting Position:

Seated or standing with arms in front of body, free or holding a pole. **Inhale**.

- **Exhale** – Lift the arms overhead.
  Inhale – Lower arms back down.

- Repeat 5-6 times.

NOTE: Keep scapula engaged on the back. Do not elevate shoulders.

FOCUS: Scapula stabilization, shoulder flexion

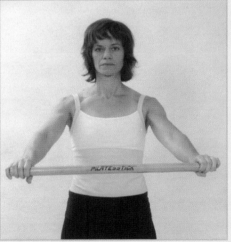

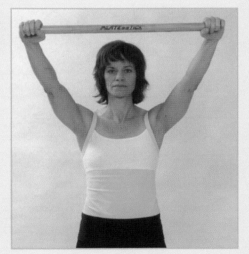

NOTES:

_____

_____

_____

13 Inner Peace Stretch

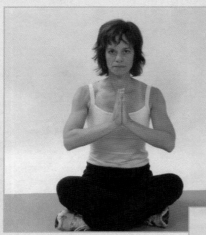

Starting Position:

Seated with the arms in front of the body, palms touching and elbows out to the side in a relaxed position. Keep arms still, but squeeze palms together, pressing into the pinkie fingers.

☙ **Inhale –** Keep palms squeezing together as you lift the arms up as high as possible.

☙ **Exhale –** Return the arms to the starting position, with the palms still squeezing together.

☙ Repeat 3-4 times.

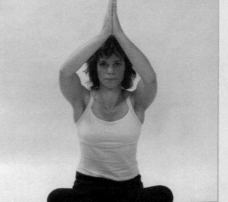

NOTE: Do not try to force the forearms/ elbows together.

FOCUS: Scapula stabilization and shoulder range of motion with core stability

NOTES:

_____

_____

_____

14 Crossing Guard

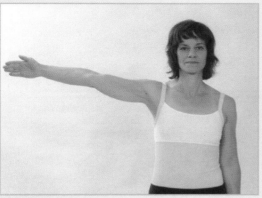

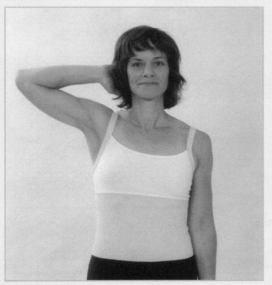

Starting Position:

Standing against a wall, both arms at your side. **Inhale**.

- **Exhale –** Using the wall as a guide, gently raise one arm out to the side (shoulder abduction), palm faces out, lifting as high as possible. At the highest range of motion, flex (bend) the elbow and try to reach behind the head. **Inhale**.

- **Exhale –** Slowly return to the start position.

- Repeat 2-3 times, then switch arms.

FOCUS: Scapula stabilization, shoulder abduction with elbow flexion

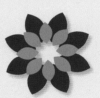

phase 3

NOTES:

_____

_____

17

15 Seated Puppet

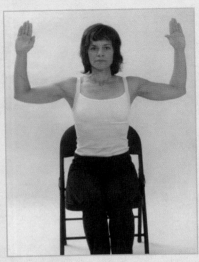

Starting Position:

Seated or standing with both arms out to the side, bend the elbows at 90 degrees, fingers pointing to the ceiling, palms facing out. **Inhale**.

- **Exhale –** Internally rotate the left arm so that the palm is facing the floor, while simultaneously externally rotating the right arm. Keep elbows open wide.

- **Inhale –** Return arms to start position, head facing forward.

- **Exhale –** Internally rotate the right arm so that the palm is facing the floor, while simultaneously externally rotating the left arm. Head rotating to the right.

- **Inhale –** Return to start position.

- Alternate 2-3 times each side.

NOTE: Your head is always turning towards the internally rotated shoulder. As you reverse arms, your head will slowly turn towards the other side.

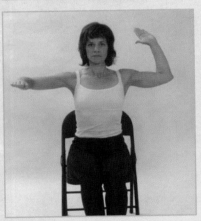

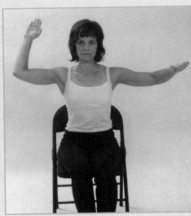

NOTES:

_____

_____

_____

16 Toe Taps

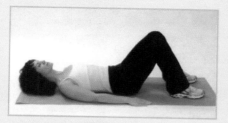

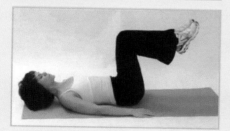

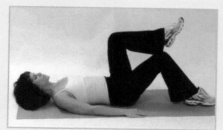

Starting Position:

Supine with knees bent and spine neutral, arms by the sides, **Inhale**. **Exhale** – Imprint the spine by lifting the hip bones up toward the rib cage.

- **Inhale** – Lift one leg up to tabletop position (create a right angle between your torso and thigh bone, and also your thigh bone and shin bone).

- **Exhale** – REALLY engage the abdominals and bring the other leg up to tabletop position as well. **Inhale** to stay.

- **Exhale** – Keeping the right angle between the thigh bone (Femur) and calf, reach one leg away and touch the toes of that foot to the ground. **Inhale** – Return leg to tabletop position. **Exhale** – Repeat with other leg.

- Alternate 5-6 times.

SPECIAL NOTE: Tramflap patients cannot stabilize in tabletop position.

NOTE: Put your thumbs on your ribs and your little fingers on your hip bones. Make sure these two points don't separate as you do this exercise.

FOCUS: Core strength and stability

NOTES:

_____

_____

_____

17 Hip Lift

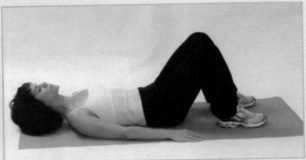

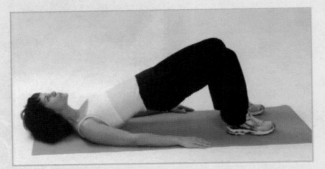

Starting Position:

Supine with knees bent and spine neutral, arms by the sides, palms down. **Inhale** to prepare.

- **Exhale** – Imagine that you are in a straight jacket and can't curl your spine. Immediately engage your gluteal muscles and abdominals and lift your hips off the floor, stopping when you have achieved a straight line between the upper rib cage and the knees. **Inhale** and hold 1-2 seconds at the top.

- **Exhale** – Keep neutral spine, and flex (bend) at the hips to lower the hips to the floor.

- Repeat 3-4 times.

NOTE: The Bridge position should be done from the hip extensors (butt & hamstrings), not from the back muscles. Keep spine in neutral; do not arch the spine.

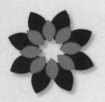

NOTES:

18 Hip Lift with Leg Lift

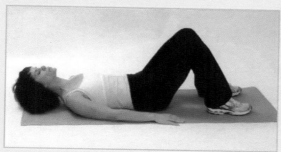

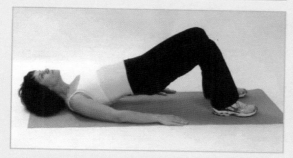

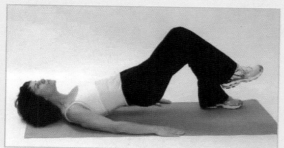

Starting Position:

Supine with knees bent and spine neutral, arms by the sides. **Inhale** to prepare.

- **Exhale –** Imagine that you are in a straight jacket and can't curl your spine. Immediately engage your gluteal muscles and abdominals and lift your hips off the floor, stopping when you have achieved a straight line between the upper rib cage and the knees. **Inhale** to stay.

- **Exhale –** Keep the neutral spine and lift your right leg 2-3 inches off the floor. Then **Inhale** to stay. **Exhale** and put your foot down.

- Repeat with the left leg. Alternate 3-4 times.

NOTES:

19 Hip Swivel with Knee Drop

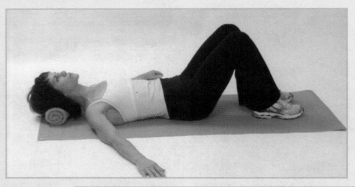

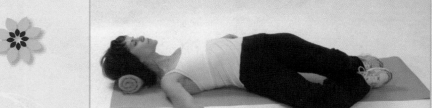

Starting Position:

Supine with knees bent and legs hip width apart. **Inhale** to prepare.

ભ **Exhale –** Keeping both shoulders on the mat, allow your knees to fall to the right side of your body. **Inhale** to stay.

ભ **Inhale –** Return to the start position.

ભ **Exhale –** Repeat on the left side.

ભ Repeat 3-4 times each side.

NOTES:

_____

_____

_____

20 Half Roll Back

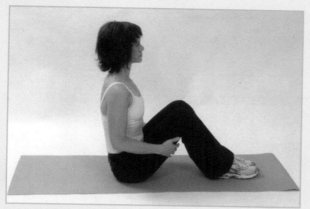

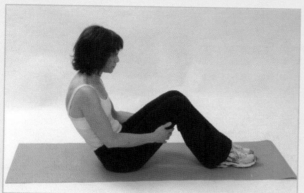

Starting Position:

Seated with the knees bent in front, feet placed on the mat, **inhale** and engage your abdominals.

☞ **Exhale –** Rounding your back, roll your spine back, off your tail bone. Create a letter "C" with your spine, feet stay on the mat. **Inhale** to stay, keeping the "C" curve.

☞ **Exhale** and roll back up to a seated position.

☞ Repeat 5-6 times.

FOCUS: Core stability and strength

NOTES:

_____

_____

21 Modified Sliding Child's Pose

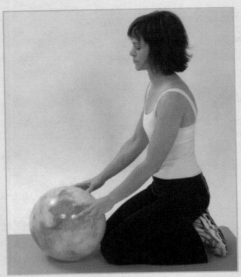

Starting Position:

On knees with arms on a ball, roller, or on the floor. **Inhale** to prepare – sit back on the backs of your legs.

❧ **Exhale** – Slide out as far as possible, feeling the stretch in the front of the chest. **Inhale**, slide back to the start position.

❧ Repeat 3-4 times.

NOTE: If you have knee problems, definitely opt for the ball. You should not sit back on your heels if you feel any pain in your knees.

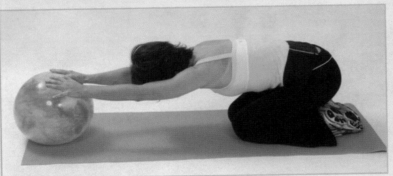

NOTES:

_____

_____

_____

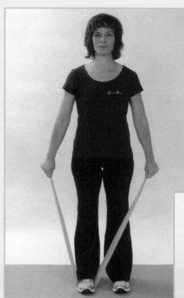

Starting Position:

Standing with the Dyna-band secured under one foot. The ends of the Dyna-band in each hand. **Inhale** to prepare.

- **Exhale –** Keeping arms straight, press arms down and back toward the hips.

- **Inhale –** Return to the start position.

- Repeat 6-8 times.

NOTE: To progress the exercise, press arms past the hip line moving into shoulder extension.

FOCUS: Scapula stabilization, shoulder range of motion

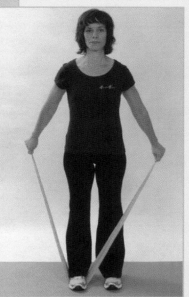

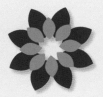

phase 4

NOTES:

23 Back Row with Dyna-band - Elbows High

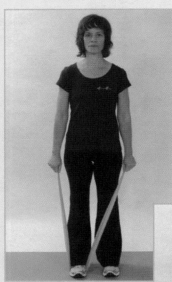

Starting Position:

Standing with the Dyna-band secure under one foot, each end of the Dyna-band in each hand. Palms facing back. **Inhale** to prepare.

> **Exhale –** Slowly bring the hands toward the body, bending elbows. As you bring the hands toward the body, try to keep elbows wide and away from the body. Keep elbows below shoulder height. Shoulder blades should move toward the spine.

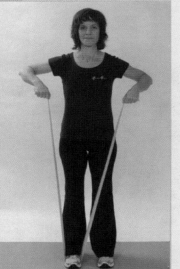

> **Inhale –** Slowly return to the start position.

> Repeat 6-8 times.

NOTE: For the Lat Flap patient, please work one arm at a time (unilateral).

FOCUS: Scapula stabilization, strengthening Latissimus Dorsi, Rhomboids

NOTES:

_____

_____

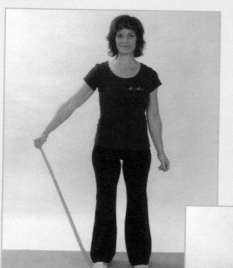

phase 4

Starting Position:

Standing with feet shoulder width apart, place one end of the Dyna-band securely under one foot, the other end in same-side hand. **Inhale** to prepare.

ℛ **Exhale –** Slowly raise the arm up and out from the side of the body until the arm is just below shoulder height.

ℛ **Inhale –** Slowly return to the start position.

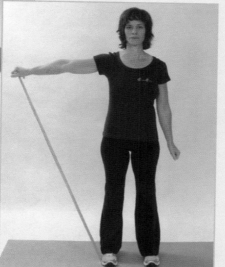

ℛ Repeat 5-6 times on each side, gradually building to 10 repetitions per side.

FOCUS:
Shoulder abduction

NOTES:

_____

_____

_____

25 Shoulder Front Raise

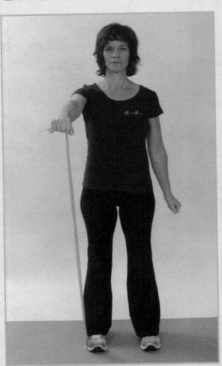

Starting Position:

Standing with feet shoulder width apart, place one end of the Dyna-band securely under one foot, the other end in same-side hand. **Inhale** to prepare.

- **Exhale –** Reach arm forward of the hip and up toward the ceiling, initiating the movement from the shoulder joint. Raise the arm to just below shoulder height.

- **Inhale –** Slowly return to the start position.

- Repeat 5-6 times on each side, gradually building to 10 repetitions per side.

FOCUS: Shoulder flexion, Scapula stabilization

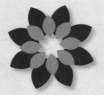

NOTES:

_____

_____

_____

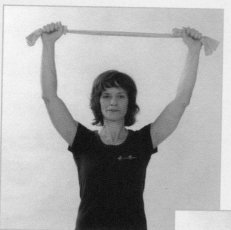

Starting Position:

Standing, grasp each end of the the Dyna-band in the right and left hands so the length of the band is shoulder width apart.

☞ **Inhale –** Extend both arms overhead.

☞ **Exhale –** Bend your torso slightly to the right. Then pull down with the right arm, keeping the left arm overhead. You can bend the right elbow if needed.

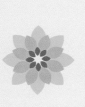

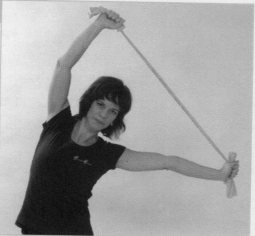

☞ **Inhale –** Release the right arm back to the overhead position and return your body to the upright position.

☞ Repeat 4-5 times each side.

NOTES:

_____

_____

27 Mermaid with Dyna-band

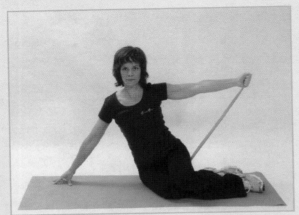

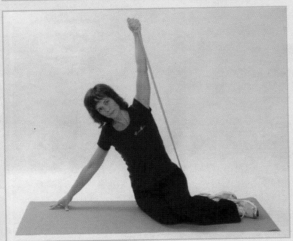

Starting Position:

Seated on the right hip with one end of the Dyna-band secured underneath you. Use your left hand to grab the other end of the Dyna-band.

- **Inhale –** Reach the left arm overhead.

- **Exhale –** Laterally flex to the right side.

- **Inhale –** Return to the upright position.

- Repeat 4-5 times on each side.

NOTES:

_____

_____

_____